TABLE OF CONTENTS

INTRODUCTION

Fit after 50 is the story of my journey from a 400 pound sickly invalid to a svelte 150 pound, healthy person.

It took me until my 58th year of life to realize that I was digging my grave with my fork (if I may borrow that cliché).

I cannot stress how much we (older people) forget that, after a certain age we cannot eat like the youngn's. I indulged my gluttonous appetite every opportunity I got. To top it off, I became very sedentary and eventually became too fat to move even if I wanted to.

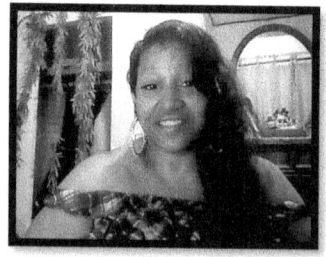

At almost 400 pounds, I never took photos below my shoulders.

Baby Boomers are one of the largest and most powerful generations in the U.S. They have redefined aging and are more educated, wealthy, and tech savvy than their parents or any generation preceding them. Yet, despite these advantages, some studies show that many Boomers are actually overweight or obese, placing them at greater risk for chronic health conditions such as heart disease, Type 2 Diabetes, and certain cancers.

Even for the most determined Baby Boomers, as we age, we often lose flexibility, strength, and balance, which makes staying, fit after 50 challenging. Working with a physical therapist, can help you address these challenges, maintain fitness, and avoid injury. While helping you achieve your fitness goals, physical therapists take an individual approach and consider any pre-existing conditions or diseases that you may have to tailor a plan that is specific to your unique needs. But it starts with YOU!

The Stats

The prevalence of obesity in the United States is increasing in all age groups. During the past 30 years, the proportion of older adults who are obese has doubled. In this article the author describes the prevalence and causes of obesity among older adults as well as the consequences of obesity in older adults. Recommendations for interventions to address obesity are also provided. In this chapter, the differences between the two groups of older adults, those 50 to 65 years of age, and those over 65 years of age, will be addressed.

Obesity is defined as abnormal accumulation of body fat, usually 20% or more over an individual's ideal body weight, is a serious and growing public health problem. The number and proportion of people who are obese have risen notably in recent decades; since the 1970s, the prevalence of obesity has more than doubled in the adult population. In 2003-2006, more than one in three adults (35.7%) were classified as obese. Overweight and obese people are more likely to have chronic health problems such as diabetes, high blood pressure, and arthritis. They also are at greater risk for developing heart disease, cancer, and Alzheimer's disease. Obesity-related health care costs in the United States were estimated to be 9.1% of total annual medical expenditures in 1998 and may have been as high as $78.5 billion ($92.6 billion in 2002 dollars). Nearly half of these costs are borne by public programs—Medicaid and Medicare.

Although Americans of all ages are increasingly overweight, policy makers and health care providers have tended to overlook the problem of obesity in middle-aged and elderly populations.

Some physicians have neglected discussing the problem with older patients, believing it too late to encourage substantive changes in their health behavior, and the media have tended to focus on obesity among children, for whom excessive weight has been a rarity until recently.

Currently, nearly one in eight Americans (12.6%) is age 65 or older. This ratio is expected to jump to one in five (19.7%) by 2030, due in part to longer life expectancies and the aging of the baby boom generation. Because the highest rates of obesity are found among baby boomers, aged 44-62 in 2008, it is likely that the prevalence of obesity among older adults will continue to climb in coming decades as this population ages. By 2010, 37.4% of adults aged 65 and older are anticipated to be obese. If this trajectory continues unabated, it is projected that nearly half of the elderly population will be obese in 2030.

Increasing levels of obesity among the elderly will be a challenging policy issue at the state and federal levels, because excessive weight gain is associated with an array of chronic conditions, and because persons with multiple chronic illnesses generate more than 65% of all Medicare costs.

To help inform Congress about patterns of weight distribution among older Americans, as well as to describe potential future trends in elderly obesity, this report presents estimates of the prevalence of obesity for adults aged 65 and older. Racial disparities in obesity and differences across age and gender lines are discussed. In addition, regional variations are presented, including state-level obesity estimates for 1995, 1999, 2003, and 2007. The report concludes with a brief description of possible policy approaches to addressing the obesity epidemic that the United States is facing.

Currently, 7% of the world's population is over 65 years of age. This figure is projected to rise to 12% by 2030. In the US it is projected to rise from 12% (35 million) to 20% (71 million) by 2030 (Yan et al., 2004). These substantial increases among older adults suggest that obesity among older Americans is likely to become a greater problem in the future (Center on an Aging Society, 2003). By 2000, the prevalence of obesity in people 50 to 69 years of age had increased to 22.9%, and for those above 70 years of age to 15%, representing increases of 56% and 36% respectively, since 1991 (Villareal et al., 2005).

Although the prevalence of obesity in persons who are over 80 years of age is about one-half that of older adults between the ages of 50 and 59, the fact is that more than 15% of the older American population is obese (Villareal et al., 2005). Moreover, as the aging population increases in number, so too will the number of chronic illnesses, which often accompany aging, increase in our society (Flood & Newman, 2007). Chronic conditions, such as arthritis, diabetes, hypertension, and heart disease, are among some of the most common, debilitating, and costly chronic conditions in older adults. These conditions are frequently accentuated by obesity (Federal Interagency Forum on Aging, 2006).

Causes of Obesity in Older Adults

An important determinant of body-fat mass is the relationship between energy intake and expenditure. Obesity occurs when a person consumes more calories than she/he burns. We need calories to sustain life and have the energy be active; yet to maintain a desirable weight, we need to balance the amount of energy we ingest in the form of food with the energy we expend (National Institutes of Health [NIH]), 2006). Weight gain occurs when the balance is tipped and we take in more calories than we burn. Most studies indicate that how much we eat does not decline with advancing age (Gary, Hunt, VanderJagt, & Vellas, 1992). Therefore it is likely that a decrease in energy expenditure, particularly in the 50- to 65-year-old age group, contributes to the increase in body fat as we age. In those 65 years of age and older, hormonal changes that occur during aging may cause the accumulation of fat. Aging is associated with a decrease in growth hormone secretions, reduced responsiveness to thyroid hormone, decline in serum testosterone, and resistance to leptin (Corpas, Harman, & Blackman, 1993). Resistance to leptin could cause a decreased ability to regulate appetite downward (Villareal et al., 2005). Genetic, environmental and social, as well as several other factors can all contribute to obesity. These factors will be discussed below.

Genetic Factors

...science does show a link between obesity and heredity. The observation, often made by nurses, that obesity tends to run in families may lead us to believe that obesity is related to the genes a person has inherited; and science does show a link between obesity and heredity (NIH, 2006). Almost 20 years ago, researchers demonstrated the role of biological inheritance in fat variations (Bouchard, 1989). Bouchard found that visceral fat is more influenced by the genotype than subcutaneous fat. It appears that a genotype-overfeeding interaction component exists for body fat, which suggests that the sensitivity of an individual to changes in body fat following overfeeding is genotype dependent. In a recently released study, researchers used structural equation modeling to identify the specific relationship between genetic loci that affect adiposity and those that affect muscle growth (Brockman, Tsaih, Neuschi, Churchill, & Li, 2008).

Environmental and Sociological Factors

Just as genetics plays a role in obesity, so does the environment. The environment includes the world around us; it influences access to healthy food and safe places to walk. What we eat, our level of physical activity, and our lifestyle behaviors are influenced by our environment. Our environment can prevent us from eating healthy foods and/or getting adequate exercise in a number of ways. Examples include the trend toward 'eating out' rather than preparing food in the home; high-fat, high-calorie foods in our workplace vending machines; neighborhoods that often lack sidewalks; and a deficit of readily accessible recreation areas.

High-calorie, processed food is less expensive and quicker to prepare than fresh fruits and vegetables. Poverty and lower levels of education have also been linked to obesity (NIH, 2006). It has been suggested that one reason why poverty and lower educational levels are risk factors for obesity is that high-calorie, processed food is less expensive and quicker to prepare than fresh fruits and vegetables (NIH, 2006). Through observation and the anecdotes patients have shared with me, I have come to believe the social environment indeed contributes to the increasing prevalence of obesity. To date, only a few research studies have focused on this factor.

Glass, Rasmussen, and Schwartz (2006) did investigate whether neighborhood psychosocial hazards, defined as "stable and visible features of neighborhood environments that give rise to a heightened state of vigilance, alarm, or fear in residents" (p. 4), independent of individual risk factors, were associated with the increased odds of obesity in older adults. After analyzing data from a cohort study of 1140 randomly selected community dwelling men and women who were 50 to 70 years of age, they found that 38% were obese. Residents living in the more hazardous neighborhoods were more than twice as likely to be obese as those living in the least-hazardous neighborhoods, even after controlling for behavioral and socioeconomic individual-level risk factors. The authors concluded that this significant finding demonstrates that neighborhood conditions can alter patterns of obesity. Community-level interventions that might lead to a reduction in environmental and sociological hazards include increasing educational attainment, increasing public safety, reducing crime rates, and eliminating vacant housing.

Other Causes of Obesity

Other conditions and illnesses that are associated with both weight gain and obesity include: hyperthyroidism, Cushing's syndrome, polycystic ovary syndrome, and depression (NIH, 2006). The older adults who are obese are more likely than those who are not obese to report symptoms of depression, such as feelings of sadness, worthlessness, and hopelessness (Center on an Aging Society, 2003). Lack of sleep may contribute to obesity, as well as certain drugs, such as steroids and some antidepressants that may stimulate the appetite, cause water retention, or slow the metabolism rate (NIH, 2008). Finally, the complex relationship between functional ability and lifestyle patterns merits attention as a contributor to obesity (Center on an Aging Society). Joint pain, decreased mobility, and activity intolerance may lead to weight gain because of decreased activity. Older adults are more likely than younger adults to experience functional limitations associated with chronic illnesses that may begin a stress-pain-depression cycle that can result in lifestyle patterns leading obesity (Lorig et al., 2006).

Consequences of Obesity in Older Adults

Health problems associated with obesity are classified as either nonfatal or life threatening by the World Health Organization (2005). This section will discuss the consequences of obesity on both nonfatal and life-threatening health problems. Interventions to address these particular consequences will be discussed as each consequence is presented. Specific interventions to decrease obesity will be discussed in the following section titled, "Interventions to Address Obesity."

Problems Related to Obesity

Debilitating conditions, such as those associated with respiratory, chronic musculoskeletal, and skin problems are classified as nonfatal, although it could be argued that any of these conditions could become life-threatening. These conditions, which are aggravated by obesity, will be discussed below.

Respiratory problems. In obese patients, lungs decrease in size. Both the increased weight on the chest wall of obese patients and the difficulty they experience in lifting the heavy chest wall may contribute to difficulty in breathing (Wallace, Schulte, Nakeeb, & Andris, 2003). Obesity is known to induce respiratory mechanical impairment that may be combined with abnormalities in gas exchange (Zerah et al., 1993). In the obese elderly, these changes are accentuated by changes in the lung structure and function associated with normal aging. These changes in the lungs include decreased alveolar surface available for gas exchange, increased chest wall stiffness, and stiffening of the elastin and the collagen tissue supporting the lungs (Tabloski, 2006). The mass loading of the ventilator system induced by obesity alters the static balance within the respiratory system. Obese older patients often have a reduced respiratory efficiency that can reach the point of respiratory insufficiency in the presence of cardiovascular insufficiency of various degrees. The natural decrease in respiratory function in older patients exacerbates the decrease caused by obesity which may in turn lead to an increase in the sleep apnea syndrome, which, in these patients, is related to a greater risk of developing hallucinatory and cognitive disorders caused by hypoxia during sleep (Donini et al., 2006).

Endurance exercise when combined with a dietary weight loss program increases maximal oxygen consumption

(Dick, 2004). Diet in conjunction with resistance and endurance exercises improves peak oxygen consumption as well. Nurses can teach patients with respiratory problems to do diaphragmatic or abdominal breathing to help strengthen respiratory muscles. Breathing exercises, as well as good posture, can help patients to exhale and inhale fully (Lorig et al., 2006). Pursed lip breathing may also be helpful for patients who are short of breath or breathless. Pursed breathing includes pursing the lips as if blowing a whistle; using diaphragmatic breathing out through pursed lips without any force; and remembering to relax the upper chest, arms shoulders, and arms while breathing out. Patients with sleep apnea need to be referred for sleep studies.

Arthritis and osteoarthritis. Arthritis is the leading cause of disability in older adults. A high body mass index (BMI) is an associated risk factor for knee osteoarthritis (OA) in older persons (Villareal et al., 2005). By 65 years of age the prevalence of osteoarthritis is 68% in women and 58% in men. This age-related increase in the prevalence of OA may reflect bodily changes as a result of a lifetime of being overweight which results in strain on weight-bearing joints (Villareal et al.).

Obesity, or even being overweight, increases the load placed on joints, especially the knee and hip joints. Breakdown in cartilage, resulting from the increased weight on joints, may result in pain and further functional disability (Lorig & Fries, 2006). Leveille, Wee, and Iezzoni (2005) reported that the relative risk of arthritis in people who are obese increases over time. People with arthritis are particularly vulnerable to the stress-pain-depression cycle mentioned above, in which the pain and stiffness caused by the disease leads to decreased mobility, thereby increasing stress, pain, and depression and likely decreasing quality of life (Newman, 2002). Obese older people above the age of 50 who have arthritis are more likely to say their condition limits their activities than non-obese adults in this age group (Center on an Aging Society, 2003).

For the older person with OA, the most important risk factor that can be modified is obesity. Karlson et al. (2003) noted during the Nurses' Health Study that of all the hip-replacement risk factors examined, including BMI, hormone replacement after menopause, alcohol use, physical activity, and cigarette smoking, only BMI and cigarette smoking were associated with needing a hip replacement.

The goal of managing arthritis is to maintain the maximum use and function of the joint and the surrounding muscles, tendons, and ligaments (Lorig et al., 2006). Exercise is the key to meeting this goal. However, many people with OA and other joint diseases believe that exercise will cause their arthritis to flare up and increase the pain. This is a misperception that nurses can work to dispel. Stretching exercises of all muscle groups should be done ten minutes a day as well as daily active range of motion for all joints. Isotonic exercises, which move the joint in an arc, are also helpful. Aquatic exercise and walking are usually well tolerated by older adults with mild to moderate lower extremity OA (Resnick, 2001). Heat is also helpful in managing arthritis because it reduces stiffness and makes exercise easier. Rest periods between activities help to control the fatigue of arthritis, which is compounded by obesity.

Although many cognitive-behavioral programs have been found to help people with arthritis manage their chronic condition, The Arthritis Self-Management Course, designed by a nurse and endorsed by the Arthritis Foundation, has been the most successful (Lorig, 2006). Nurses can make referrals to this program, or become self-management course leaders. Many of the interventions described in the upcoming section on Interventions for Obesity in Older Adults also apply to those having OA.

Skin conditions. Brown, Wimpenny, and Maughan (2004) found skin problems, including itching, skin breakdown, redness, and rashes, in 75% of the obese population they sampled. The two main causes of the reported skin problems were perspiration and friction. Groin, limbs, and under breasts were identified as the most troubling areas. Older adults who are obese and have skin problems face additional complications because their skin naturally loses about 20% of its dermal thickness with age (Baranoski, 2001). This combination of older age, fragile skin, and obesity increases the risk for pressure sores (Flood & Newman, 2007).

The first step in addressing skin problems is to conduct a skin assessment of obese patients. The specificity and degree of skin problems will determine the intervention. Nurses are advised to initiate measures to decrease friction as soon as possible after hospital admission. Additionally, in older women, urinary incontinence from a large, heavy abdomen causing the valve on the bladder to weaken may result in the leaking of urine when coughing or sneezing. Nurses should educate patients about keeping the area dry so as to prevent skin problems. Strategies to keep the area dry include wearing absorption pads in their underwear and changing underwear as soon as possible when leakage occurs.

Life-Threatening Illnesses Related to Obesity

The World Health Organization (2005) has noted that life-threatening illnesses related to obesity include cardiovascular disease; conditions associated with insulin resistance, such as type 2 diabetes; certain types of cancers, especially hormonally related and large-bowel cancer; and gallbladder disease. The next few sections will discuss these illnesses.

Cardiovascular disease. Coronary heart disease is responsible for significant morbidity and mortality in older patients who are 65 years and older. It remains a leading cause of mortality in the US with 84% of persons 65 years or older dying from this disease (Hanna & Wenger, 2005).

Dietary modification is the cornerstone of treating cardiovascular disease in older adults who are obese. Grundy (2004) has described obesity as a major underlying factor contributing to atherosclerotic cardiovascular disease (ASCVD) and a factor associated with multiple other ASCVD risk factors, including elevated blood pressure, hypertriglyceridemia, low high-density lipoproteins, high cholesterol, and high fasting plasma glucose. It is also a risk factor for type 2 diabetes. Even though there is a strong association between obesity and ASCVD, the relationship underlying the mechanism is not well understood. The fact that obesity acts on so many metabolic pathways, producing so many potential risk factors, makes it challenging to delineate the specific mechanism by which obesity contributes to ASCVD. Gundy suggested that the fundamental question for controlling cardiovascular diseases related to obesity is: how can we intervene at the public health level to reduce the high prevalence of obesity in the general population. He added that indeed, "This approach offers the greatest possibility for reducing the cardiovascular risk that accompanies obesity" (p. 2600). The widely disseminated Healthy People 2010 (U.S. Department of Health and Human Services, n.d.) challenges individuals, communities, professionals, and indeed all of us, to take specific steps to reduce obesity to ensure that good health, as well as long life, are enjoyed by all. Dietary modification is the cornerstone of treating cardiovascular disease in older adults who are obese. Interventions to decrease obesity are presented in the next section titled, "Interventions to Address Obesity."

Diabetes. Type 2 diabetes, the most common type of diabetes in older adults, results from interplay between genetic factors and environmental factors that contribute to

25

obesity. Even a 15 pound weight gain can increase a person's risk of diabetes by 50% (Daniels, 2006). There is an age-related increase in total body fat and visceral adiposity until age 65 that is often accompanied by diabetes or impaired glucose intolerance (Wilson & Kannel, 2007). In the Framingham Study 30-40% of people over 65 were found to have diabetes or glucose intolerance. Coronary disease is the most common and lethal sequel of type 2 diabetes. Lean-muscle mass begins to diminish after the age of 65. This decrease may be related to decreased physical activity, disability, anabolic hormone production, or increased cytokine activity. If calorie intake continues at the same rate while the muscle mass decreases, the older person will most likely experience fat weight gain (Tucker, 2006).

The chief goal for obese diabetic persons is to avoid the common cardiovascular sequelae (Wilson & Kannel, 2007). The effect of sedentary behavior, particularly television watching, in relation to risk of type 2 diabetes was studied by a group of researchers who followed a cohort of subjects from the Nurses' Health Study (Hu, Li, Colditz, Willett, & Manson, 2003). These researchers reported that time spent watching TV was positively associated with risk of obesity and type 2 diabetes. Each two-hour-a-day increment in watching TV was associated with a 23% increase in obesity and a 14% increase in risk of diabetes. As with heart disease, a comprehensive approach to social and environmental factors, including weight reduction is suggested. Specific dietary modifications are suggested in the next section, "Interventions to Address Obesity."

Cancer. Obesity is also linked to higher rates of certain types of cancer (NIH, 2006). Breast cancer in older women is increasingly being linked to obesity (Sweeney, Blair, Anderson, Lazovich, & Folsom, 2004). Twenty-five to 30% of several major cancers, including breast (postmenopausal), colon, kidney, and esophageal, have been linked to obesity and physical inactivity (Vainio & Bianchini, 2002). Men who are obese are more likely to develop cancer of the colon, rectum, or prostate, than men who are not obese. Cancer of the gallbladder, uterus, cervix, or ovaries are more common in women who are obese compared with women who are not obese (NIH, 2006). Management of obesity is needed to decrease the incidence of these cancers.

Gallbladder disease. Obesity is a major risk factor for gallstones because obesity is believed to reduce the amount of bile salts in bile, resulting in more cholesterol. Additionally, gallbladder emptying is decreased as a result of obesity (National Digestive Diseases Clearinghouse, 2004). Again, management of obesity, as described below, is the primary approach for decreasing the incidence of this gallbladder disease.

Get a Life!

These **10 Quick Tips** can help you get a renewed passion for life:

1. Renew Your Faith

God is the only one who can make and KEEP you healthy, not your doctor and certainly not you. Healthy people die every day. Without spiritual grounding, you are living everyday on borrowed time. If you get sick, your doctor can assist you, but all healing comes from God. Even when surgery is involved, the outcome is much more dependent on God's will than it is your surgeon's skill. The surgeon makes the healing 'possible' but it is God who guides the scalpel.

2. Retirement is around the corner

Don't be one of those old folks who leave their retirement party feeling like someone died. Long before you retire you need to find your passion and make it a part of your life so that when you retire you can totally immerse yourself in it. When you start following your passion, magical things happen. You will find your energy increases. You will find that as soon as you awaken you JUMP out of bed excited to start the day. Your mood improves too, you sleep better, and you are generally fired up about life. If your passion is collecting Barbie Dolls then get started NOW. Read everything you can about your hobby, works on becoming the world's #1 expert, join clubs, build a website. Who knows, your passion might end up making money so that you can retire early and get paid doing what you love.

3. Volunteer – Do something for others

If you ever find yourself feeling sorry for yourself you need to drop whatever you are doing and volunteer ASAP. If you think YOU have problems; try volunteering at a VA hospital, homeless shelter or AIDS hospice and it will put your problems in the proper perspective. The volunteers often seem to get just as much or more out of the charity than the people being helped. Think outside the box and find something that takes advantage of your unique talents. It would be wonderful if you could use your unique gift to bring joy and light to others. I often donate my books to those who cannot afford to purchase them (i.e., the homeless). If you are a plumber, consider volunteering for Habitat for Humanity. Whatever knowledge you have, think of a unique way to share it. If you cannot think of anything; try volunteering at the local animal shelter.

4. Read to keep your brain engaged

Reading is a great for many reasons but mainly because it makes you think. It exposes you to wonderful and unique ideas you have never thought of. It keeps your brain young. It can be an excellent component of a stress reduction plan. Read whatever you want (preferably my books…smile), it can be "brain-candy" or highly intellectual – whatever suits your mood. Don't read what you think will be good for you because then it becomes a chore, read what you *want* to read so it's fun! If reading really isn't your thing, find something cerebral that works for you (noooooot video games): crossword puzzles, Sudoku, chess, or whatever but you activity you are able to do that causes your brain to go into overdrive.

5. Find a sport

Hopefully you have a sport you love by now but if not you need to find one. It doesn't matter what it is as long as you love it: shuffleboard, hiking, cricket, golf, skiing, biking, skating, dancing, or even horseshoes. If you already have a sport you love, it might be time to think of a more age appropriate one. Skateboarding is fun in your 30s and 40s but it's probably not advisable for 70 year olds; so you may want to rethink that one.

6. Diet – Eat unprocessed food

- FIRST drink water like a fish

- SECOND eat vegetables like a rabbit

- THIRD eat whole grains like a horse

- FOURTH eat only lean cuts of chicken

- FIFTH eat fresh fruits

- SIXTH ELIMINATE fast food and junk food

7. Make cardio part of your daily life!

Over age 50, cardiovascular health is most peoples #1 problem – make daily cardio part of your daily activity. If you have never done daily cardio then you need to get a dog, TODAY, and you need to walk it twice a day. Having a dog is a great way to force you to do your daily cardio and if you haven't established a solid habit of daily cardio by age 50 then you NEED to be forced and a dog is a perfect way. Not only do pet owners live longer, happier lives but by adopting a dog from the local shelter you are choosing a friend for life as these are some of the most loyal dogs on the planet.

8. Throw away your alarm clock

Throw out that alarm clock! Alarms are a poor solution to a time management problem.

In my opinion alarm clocks only serve one purpose and that is to wake you up before you have had enough sleep! Sleep deprivation has many, many problems associated with it. Reduced reaction times, increased stress levels, decreased ability to concentrate, increased body fat. So, what to do...well that leads me to my next point...

9. Put important things FIRST

Prayer is important so do that first. Sleep is also important so go to bed about 12 hours before you have to be to work and don't set an alarm. When you wake up naturally and then begin your day's tasks with the most important first.

You have precious little time left in this world, make the time count. Do a time audit to see if you are truly spending your time on the important things. Just for one day, keep a 'timecard' and 'charge' every activity down to the 0.1 hour. Is spending an hour on Facebook every day really that important? Will the earth stop rotating if you don't clean your house weekly? Is spending an hour watching the news a priority when you can read it in 5 minutes? How important is watching those three reality shows that you love? Please read one of my favorite books, The Manipulation of America. In this book, (written by yours truly and available on Amazon) you will see how television is used to manipulate your everyday life. Once you get up from in front of the tell-lies-vision I assure you that you will begin spending more time on the things that matter MOST to YOU.

10. Take control of health

Don't blindly do what the doctor says. Always weigh the pros and cons and make your own decisions. Remember that doctors need to make money. Invasive test aren't always in your best health interest. Take CAT scans for example, these expose you to hundreds of times the radiation of an x-ray and increase your risk of cancer. If your doctor recommends a CAT scan, ask them why, what they expect to learn, and how their treatment of you will vary depending on the outcome of the test. It's your body and you need to decide if the benefit of the test or procedure is worth the risks. If your doctor can't explain the risks and benefits clearly, find another doctor and get a second opinion. If your doctor tries to bully or intimidate you into doing something you are uncomfortable doing with the *"If you don't do this you have to sign a waiver because I cant be responsible for your death"* then find a new doctor. A great example of how to do this is the case of 85 year-old Helen. Ten years ago after she had a cancerous polyp removed from her colon. The doctor said there was a 95% chance that he got it all but she STILL needed to do chemotherapy. Helen replied *"no way!"* She explained that she was 85 years old and that the diminished quality of life from the chemotherapy wasn't worth it considering there was a 95% chance she was fine. Her doctor respected her decision and she is now a healthy 95 years old – who knows what problems might have happened had she done chemo.

Stress: Try exercise instead of medication

Sleep: Try prayer and meditation instead medication

Joint and back pain: Try exercise instead of surgery

High Cholesterol: Try a change in diet instead of medication.

GOING THROUGH THE "CHANGES"

Fashion is NOT always your friend. Fashionable YES...foolish NOOOOO! If a woman is pushing 40 she only looks desperate by wearing a mini skirt or biker shorts; no matter how great her figure is. Nothing looks worse than mutton dressed like lamb.

Don't compare your life to others'. You have no idea what their journey is all about.

While you walk, smile. It is the ultimate antidepressant

Hug at least 8 times a day

You don't have to win every argument. Agree to disagree.

Live with the 3 E's

Energy, Enthusiasm, & Empathy

Ladies - burn those 'special' scented candles, use the 600 or higher thread count sheets, the good china and wear our fancy lingerie now. Stop waiting for a special occasion. Every day is special.

Keep it simple. Be wary of get-rich-quick schemes or sales pitches for complex investments, such as oil-and-gas partnerships, that trade on the millionaire cachet to lure investors into buying high-fee products they don't understand. Most millionaire households accumulate their wealth over the long term by sticking to a regular investing plan in a balanced portfolio

Create a professional-looking page on Myspace, Facebook, Twitter, Linkin, etc., that tells folks what you are all about, and don't neglect more conventional networking: Join a professional association or show up at school reunions and after work events toting business cards.

Contribute as much as you can to your 401(k) and other tax-deferred retirement plans. You'll not only build a bigger nest egg, but you'll also cut your tax bill. In the 25% federal tax bracket, every $1,000 you contribute to a 401(k) trims your taxes by $250. And you'll save on state income taxes, too.

Do not take pictures with drinks in your hands or hold up the peace sign...ugh

Tricks to STAYING young

If the 50's are the new 40...well then you should look 37...

- Rubber sole shoes scream old lady. Wear heels or flat sexy sandals; anywhere from 1 inch to 4inches
- Groom your eyebrows
- Buy new bras that fit
- If you have rolls or you have side/front and back muffin tops that are visible over your pants, shorts, or skirt; steer clear of tight clothing.

- Invest in Shapewear

- Sit up straight and you appear to lose 3-5lbs.

- Wear more dresses

- No white or nude stockings

- Use African Shea Butter to decrease the appearance of cellulite & soften stretch marks

- Update your jewelry

- Use lady speed stick CLINCAL PROOF to eliminate white residue on underarm skin and clothing.

- Buy Quality clothes

- Brighten your teeth

- ***Drink green tea and plenty of water.***

- Eat Alaskan salmon broccoli, almonds& walnuts.

- Smile and laugh more.

Fit Women over 50

KHANDI ALEXANDER

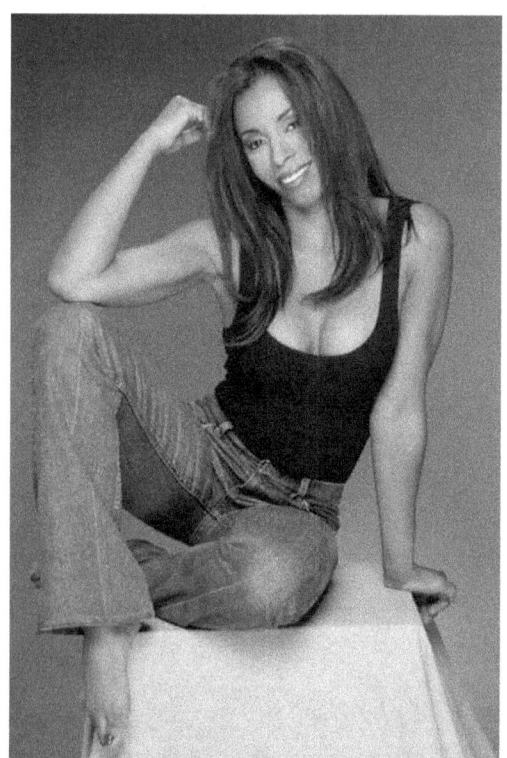

Age: 55

Accomplishment: One of my favorite actresses, Khandi Alexander is an American dancer, choreographer, and film and television star. She is perhaps best known for the roles of Dr. Alexx Woods on CSI: Miami and as Catherine Duke on NewsRadio.

ERNESTINE SHEPHERD

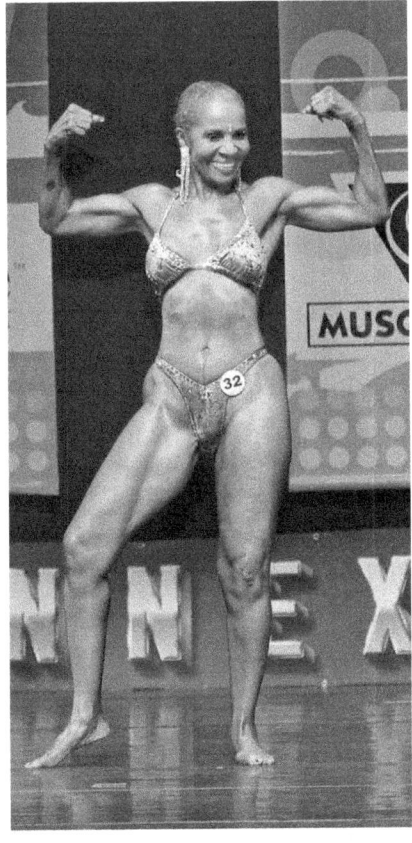

Age: 76

Accomplishment: Mrs. Shepherd shows us time and time again that age is just a number and you can achieve your goals if you are willing to put in the work to get them. More importantly, she shows us that you can benefit tremendously from regular exercise both physically and mentally. When you increase blood flow in the body through exercise, you increase blood flow to the brain which is beneficial in preventing dementia and Alzheimer's disease. (Source: Senior Journal.com.)

Christie Brinkley

Age: 58

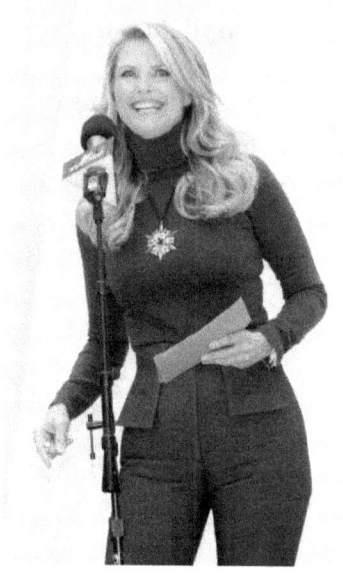

Christie Brinkley has had the longest running contract of any model ever with *CoverGirl*. She my favorite uptown girl. She's currently on Broadway, promoting skincare and more. To keep a schedule like hers, she has to stay in shape.

So if you thought that age would stop you from being who you want to be, hopefully looking at these fabulous old gals has changed your mind.

Another P.O.V. on Aging

Despite how great we can make ourselves look and feel; I have bad news for you. For many, fifty is <u>not</u> the new 40; **50 is 50**. Fifty is the end of youth. There is no escape from Planet Fifty; it is inhabited by middle-aged people, by people who, for the most part, don't look young any more.

Someone has to say it. And besides, it's the truth. Sure 50-somethings can dress up the situation - teeth whitening, hair plugs, liposuction, cool clothes - and convince one another that they're actually living on a younger planet, but they're not.

It's a bit sad really.

Why are baby boomers so obsessed with aging? Could it be that beyond 50 (for that's where boomers are) it's all downhill. No, there isn't a plateau in this decade; no, there isn't a secret passage that pops you back to 33; no, the whole decade slopes in one irreversible gravity-induced direction. Fifty leads to 60 and then on to the great abyss which is 70 and beyond. (Whispers): *I have never heard of anyone returning from the abyss.* Apart from the odd Hollywood actor or actress no one looks good beyond 50. Or at least no one natural, that is.

Baby boomers like me who have had only two or less kids and went to the gym well into our 40s and don't eat carbs deserve to look 50 when we are 60. Or perhaps even 45 in the dim lighting...right or at the very least from a distance.

So sixty is the new 40, 70 is the new 50, 110 is the new 108, etc. It means that people are living longer today, they're healthier, and they're enjoying life more. All that is great. However, at the same time that people are feeling much younger than people their age felt in previous generations, an all-powerful culture of youth is dominating our society. People in their 20s are getting cosmetic surgery to look younger. Men and women in their 40s are considered too old to work in some fields. More and more people are forced to take early retirement at an earlier and earlier age. So while older people are feeling younger these days, our society may be seeing them as older, not younger. Maybe in terms of perceptions, 40 is the new 60.

Today, the average age for someone moving into a nursing home is 81. In the 1950's, it was 65. In a 2005 Merrill Lynch survey of people between the ages of 40 and 59, 76 percent said they planned to retire when they were about 64 — and then start an entirely new career. Men and women in their 70s and 80s race in almost every marathon. Seniors teach and take classes, travel, and just seem to live fuller lives than ever before.

But that's not how society sees them. Judging by TV commercials, right when we get out of baby diapers, we have to prepare ourselves to get into adult diapers. And look how young the people are in the ads for Viagra-like products, hair dyes, and arthritis medications. It's as if

Madison Avenue is saying that it's over for you once you're past the grand old age of 25.

There is one area in our society in which being older is not held against you. And it's the one area that maybe it should be — presidential politics. Being young can actually hurt a candidate. We hear things like, "Is he too inexperienced?" or "Is he mature enough?" The majority of today's candidates are too old to be considered for most jobs in the "real world." But apparently, Americans like their leaders to look like parents, or grandparents. It's ironic that just when people might be getting a bit more forgetful, when they may have a few more health problems, when they have less and less of a connection to America's youth, that's when they are considered the right age to lead our country.

But for the rest of the population, ageism is a problem. People employed in television and other fields no longer worry about being blacklisted. But they fear being "gray-listed." If you're lucky enough to still work at your job after

20 or 30 years, those young people who roll their eyes when you start talking about how things were done "back in the old days" are the same people who want your job — and will probably get it. The best comeback I ever heard in reply to "that was in your day" came from a wonderful woman named Mary Braswell who would always retort, *"It's STILL my day, I haven't gone yet."* My sentiments exactly…

Despite those who *hate* on us old folk; there is STILL hope and HELP if you want it….

Seeking Help

Life at Brookhaven

On July 3rd I was swollen to TWICE my original size. Instead of the barbecue I had intended to be at the following day; I found myself a patient on Beth Israel's Cardiac ward. I was told in the ER, had I waited another day, they would have been wheeling me to the morgue instead a ward. I stayed in the hospital for one week following a diagnosis of Type 2 Diabetes and high blood pressure. From the hospital, I was sent to a physical rehabilitation facility for 21 days to unlearn my lifelong food habits and to receive intensive physical therapy. I am so thankful to God for sparing me.

I pulled up to the doors of Brookhaven in the back of a private ambulette.

I was put in the semi-private room with A.L., a cantankerous old gal who weighed about 400 pounds and looked like the actor, Peter O'Toole. Although all of the rooms had individual televisions, there was a lounge on every floor equipped with oversized furniture and a color TV. The main dining room was also the site of the recreational activities. It had a large screen TV, and the rec staff hosted parties, movies, games, musical shows, discussion groups, and more.

The Program

The Bariatric Wellness Program at Brookhaven Rehabilitation and Health Care Center supports the theory that morbid obesity is a chronic disease. Keeping this in mind the program has been designed to assist overweight residents in achieving their goal of weight loss, rehabilitation, and eventual return to independent living in the community.

The Wellness Program has developed a treatment model which is an interdisciplinary centered approach with a common goal of lifestyle change and functional independence. Each resident is required to actively participate in their plan of care which is structured around education to learn lifestyle change in order to achieve weight loss in a way that facilitates long term results, as well as to maintain the highest practicable physical, mental, and psychosocial well-being.

A multi-disciplinary team of specialists in nutrition, physical therapy, occupational therapy, psychotherapy, medicine} and nursing coordinate efforts to provide the residents with individualized care.

Promoting Recovery and Independence

Residents receive intensive physical and occupational therapy to assist in activities of daily life, strengthening techniques, ambulation, balance, climbing steps and transfer training. Our goal is to assist residents in becoming as mobile as possible, to regain independence and enjoy a more fulfilling life when they return to the community.

Residents often enter our program with multiple medical problems common among obese persons. Diagnoses may include: cardiovascular disease such as congestive heart failure or stroke, diabetes, hypertension, cellulitis, lymphodema, or osteoarthritis.

Facing Fears

We understand that one of those most painful aspects of obesity is the emotional suffering it causes the residents and their families. We place a strong emphasis on individual, group and family counseling to assist residents in their recovery by building self-esteem and confidence to overcome embarrassment, frustration, loneliness, isolation, and depression.

Overcoming Obstacles

Residents participate in some form of daily psychotherapy with our full-time social works. These valuable methods of communication, validation, camaraderie and support provide residents with the tools they need to return home with strength, determination and the goal of maintaining a healthy, productive life. Weekly "community meetings" encourage continued communication between participants and staff who meet to discuss the program.

Healthy Eating... An Essential Ingredient for Successful Recovery

Brookhaven's full-time dietitians created and planned healthy menus, teaching residents the dynamics of good nutrition, label analysis and the importance of a healthy diet. My therapeutic diet (per my diabetes diagnosis) was easily accommodated avoiding rich and unhealthy foods.

Exercising Mind and Body

A major focus of Brookhaven's rehabilitation program was to introduce exercise as an enjoyable and critical part of everyday life for residents as they move toward a healthier lifestyle. The exercise program seeks to increase energy level, decrease appetite, preserve muscle mass during weight loss, reduce body fat, increase flexibility, improve motor coordination and promote ambulation and activity

The daily recreation program, including evening activities, provided a wide range of activities including computer access, playing the card game *Spades* (my personal favorite) movies, exercise groups, happy hour and entertainment to promote recovery.

Rehabilitation, Recovery and Return to Home

Discharge planning was also an integral part of the rehabilitation process. The staff worked with me to make the transition home as safe and successful as possible.

Overall, the majority of the staff was committed to providing the highest professional level of quality care.

On July 26, 2013, I walked out of **Brookhaven Rehabilitation Facility** 50 pounds lighter and ready to resume my life.

ℰ⌘⅋

Brookhaven Rehab & Health Care Center

250 Beach 17th Street
Far Rockaway, NY 11691

Phone: 718-471-7500
Fax: 718-327-9074

ℰ⅋

Interventions to Address Obesity

As care providers for older adults, nurses are in a position to assist older adults who are obese in adopting changes to promote a healthier lifestyle. The primary goal is to achieve sustained lifestyle changes through dietary modifications, exercise, and use of community supports (Villareal et al., 2005). Strategies that promote lifestyle modifications include helping older adults who are obese to overcome barriers related to dietary changes and physical activity. Two well-developed programs, as well as general considerations to facilitate safe dietary changes and safe increases in physical activity, will be discussed below.

The Chronic Disease Self-Management Program

The Chronic Disease Self-Management Program has been developed by Kate Lorig, a nurse, and her colleagues at Stanford University. While this program is not directed specifically at obese older adults, it has been used to help people with heart disease, arthritis, diabetes, and respiratory problems learn to self-manage their conditions through increasing their self-efficacy. It develops confidence in one's ability to make the changes needed to lead a healthier life style through having participants make an action plan for each week. Each action plan addresses the questions of: what, how much, when, how often, and how confident older adults are that they can carry out the plan. Research has demonstrated that on a scale of one to ten (with ten being the most confident), people who rate themselves as at least a seven are more likely to be able to make the changes to become a more positive self-manager of their chronic condition than are those who score lower on the scale (Lorig et al, 2006). This program can be used as a prototype for nurses helping obese older adults to achieve success in losing weight.

The National Blueprint

Doctors, nutritionists and caregivers can assist clients to identify physical activity options that match their interests, lifestyles, and functional abilities; and identify opportunities for them to pursue these activities. The National Blueprint (n.d.) is a guide for organizations, associations, and agencies to help adults 50 years and older to increase their physical activity. This document synthesizes input from more than 65 individuals, representing 48 organizations, including the American College of Sports Medicine, the American Heart Association, and the National Institute on Aging (National Blueprint). The Blueprint addresses the barriers to increasing physical activity among older adults. It outlines suggestions related to addressing home and community, policy and advocacy, research, and other cross-cutting issues to overcome these barriers. Strategies in which nurses can be involved include:

Disseminating information about the benefits of physical activity in older adults to health professionals via professional journals, professional societies, and professional meetings.

Assisting clients to identify physical activity options that match their interests, lifestyles, and functional abilities; and identify opportunities for them to pursue these activities.

Providing health professionals with resources describing physical activity opportunities for the older population so professionals can make referrals and recommendation as appropriate.

The National Blueprint is available online in a printer-friendly version at <www.agingblueprint.org/>. It is an excellent resource for clinical practice as well as for generating ideas and plans for community service opportunities (Flood & Newman, 2007).

Safe Weight Loss Strategies

Older persons present special challenges when making changes in diet and activity levels. In patients over 65, the increase in chronic diseases associated with aging reduces physical activity and exercise capacity, making it more difficult for elderly persons to lose weight. Widowhood, loneliness, isolation, and depression are other factors that need to be addressed during weight-loss programs (Villareal et al., 2005). Participation in these programs by family members, as well as caregiver(s) is especially important if the older person's vision and hearing are impaired or if there is cognitive impairment.

Appropriate nutritional counseling through referral to a registered dietitian is recommended to ensure that the older adult's daily nutritional requirements are met during weight-loss programs. The benefits and risks of weight reduction in older adults should be carefully considered. Loss of lean body mass, which is already diminished in older adults, may not be appropriate in persons over 65 years of age because the loss of fat-free mass in older adults is associated with significant morbidity and mortality (Flood & Newman, 2007). A weight loss program that minimizes muscle and bone loss is recommended for the older adult who is obese and who has functional impairments or metabolic complications that might be improved by weight loss (Villareal et al., 2005). This is best achieved through a moderate reduction in daily calorie intake (500-750 kcal/d). Appropriate nutritional counseling through referral to a registered dietitian is recommended to ensure that the older adult's daily nutritional requirements are met during weight-loss programs. It is important that the diet continue to contain 1.0g/kg of protein and include 1500mg Ca/d, as well as 1000 IU vitamin D/d (Villareal et al.).

Improving physical function and helping to preserve muscle and bone mass through regular physical exercise is important in older adults who are obese. Increasing flexibility, endurance, and strength are the goals of regular exercise in older adults who are obese. Stretching, aerobic, and strengthening exercises are recommended by the American Society for Nutrition and the North American Association for the Study of Obesity and the Obesity Society, even for very old or frail persons (Villareal et al., 2005). To avoid musculoskeletal injuries and encourage adherence, exercise should be started at a low intensity and gradually progress over several weeks or months to a more vigorous level.

About Weight Loss Surgery

The increasing girth of people in the United States (US) is evident at every turn. Recall your last trip to the store, out to dinner, to the park, or at work, and ask yourself how many overweight people you observed on these occasions. While the statistics related to overweight and obese children and adults are no longer shocking, they do continue to be quite worrisome. It is unfortunate that what we truly know about obesity is sparse in comparison to the rate at which it is spreading. While energy balance is certainly an important factor in weight management, only recently have we come to appreciate that obesity is really a very complex disease that involves a wide variety of factors, including metabolic, environmental, social, behavioral, and psychological factors.

As the prevalence of obesity sky rockets worldwide, the search for successful weight- management strategies follows. For select individuals, surgical intervention is the most appropriate weight-management intervention for sustained weight loss. Surgical procedures, such as the Roux-en-Y gastric bypass, sleeve gastrectomy, and laparoscopic adjustable gastric banding, bring about both dramatic weight loss and the ability to provide the patient with marked improvement in obesity-related conditions such as diabetes, arthritis, hypertension, and obstructive sleep apnea.

The association of obesity with chronic diseases, such as heart disease, hypertension, sleep apnea, degenerative joint disease, gastroesophageal reflux disease, asthma, and depression, is well documented and reinforces the benefit of achieving and maintaining a "normal" weight.

he U.S. Department of Health and Human Services (DHHS) National Institutes of Health (NIH) Clinical Guidelines (1998) addressing weight-loss surgery indicate that surgery is an appropriate option, and poses an acceptable operative risk, for people who have a BMI>40, or BMI >35 with along with comorbid conditions, such as cardiovascular disease, sleep apnea, uncontrolled type 2 diabetes, and/or physical problems interfering with performance of daily activities. Additional criteria include failure of medically supervised, nonsurgical weight-loss programs; absence of uncontrolled psychotic or depressive disorders; and absence of current alcohol or substance abuse. The ideal candidate is highly motivated, well-informed, and has a supportive family and social environments.

Preoperative Evaluation

Once the patient qualifies for surgery, a thorough preoperative assessment takes place to optimize the patient's health status, reduce operative risk, and identify potential barriers to the desired outcome. Depending on the patient's health status, this process may take several weeks to several months. In the first step, the patient completes a comprehensive questionnaire that provides the bariatric team, consisting of surgeons, dietitians, psychologists, nurses, and bariatricians (physicians who specializes in the medical management of weight loss), a "snapshot" of the patient's lifestyle. Included are questions about medical, surgical, and psychological history, food intake and eating habits, activities of daily living, mobility, and activity tolerance.

The next step is a detailed physical exam by the surgeon which may prompt further evaluation by specialists in the areas of cardiology, pulmonology, endocrinology, anesthesia, or vascular medicine. In anticipation of surgery, specialists adjust treatment regimes for the most effective management of chronic conditions, thereby optimizing the patient's physical status. The patient also completes a battery of diagnostic tests that establish baseline values and examine preoperative function. Included are the assessment of complete blood counts, electrolytes, renal and hepatic function, chest x-ray, and electrocardiography. In patients with known heart disease and poor exercise tolerance a dobutamine stress echocardiography may be required.

The psychologist also meets with the patient to assess general competency; readiness for change; commitment to weight loss; mental status; the presence of substance abuse, including tobacco; and/or an underlying eating disorder, such as binge eating. The patients are required to quit smoking prior to surgery. I find this interesting considering that overeating is also an addiction which the surgery will not "cure." A few of the most common procedures are:

Laparoscopic Adjustable Gastric Band

The surgical procedures most commonly performed today work on two principles: restriction and malabsorption. Procedures, such as the laparoscopic adjustable gastric band (LAGB), and the laparoscopic sleeve gastrectomy (LSG) are successful simply because they restrict the amount of food the patient is able to consume at any one meal without interfering with digestion. Laparoscopic gastric banding has gained favor in that it is the least invasive of the restrictive procedures. It results in early and prolonged satiety, it is adjustable, and it is fully reversible. An inflatable gastric band is placed around the upper stomach creating a small gastric pouch and a narrow outlet to the stomach.

Roux-en-y Gastric Bypass

The Roux-en-y (rü-en-wi) (RNYGBP) gastric bypass is a procedure that employs both mechanisms of restriction and malabsorption to achieve weight loss. Food intake is limited by dividing the stomach to create a 15-30 ml pouch which is then connected to a loop of small intestine. Connecting the gastric pouch to the small intestine allows food to bypass the distal stomach, duodenum, and a portion of the jejunum, thus achieving malabsorption.

The keys to preventing post-operative complications for the bariatric-surgery patient are also a careful and thorough baseline assessment and close surveillance. The customary postoperative nursing measures, specifically pain management, wound care, venous thromboembolism prophylaxis, pulmonary toilet, early and frequent ambulation, line and drain maintenance, fluid balance, nutrition therapy, continued education, and emotional support, are of paramount importance.

Complications

Typical postoperative complications include hemorrhage, surgical-site infection, sepsis, atelectasis, and pulmonary embolism. Complications directly related to bariatric-surgery procedures are divided into two categories, namely early complications and late complications. Of the early complications (those occurring prior to hospital discharge), one of the most serious is an anastomotic or staple-line leak.

As intraperitoneal irritation progresses, patient presentation is characterized by complaints of increasing pain, hiccups, restlessness, and tachycardia. The condition of the patient with a leak may rapidly deteriorate as peritonitis, sepsis, and respiratory distress ensue. Therefore, any element of suspicion (tachycardia, fever, tachypnea, oliguria, or increasing oxygen requirement) warrants a call to the surgeon in anticipation of orders for gastrografin swallow x-ray, computed tomography scan with contrast, and/or a return trip to the operating room. Who needs that?

Personally I don't recommend getting weight loss surgery. I have heard far too many instances of folks who got the surgery and then proceeded to gain back all, if not more of their lost weight due to an inability to put the fork down.

Conclusion

The number of obese Americans ages 65 and older will increase from 10.3 million to 14.3 million by 2010, averaging 400,000 new obese adults per year (Arteburn, Crane, & Sullivan, 2004). Today, more than 65% of adults in the United States are overweight or obese. Obesity puts people at risk for heart disease, type 2 diabetes, high blood pressure, stroke, and some types of cancer.

In patients over 65, the increase in chronic diseases associated with aging reduces physical activity and exercise capacity, making it more difficult for elderly persons to lose weight. The large number of older people with obesity and associated serious health risks make understanding the causes of obesity crucial. Obese older adults are more likely to be severely disabled and require the assistance of another person than those who are not obese (Center on an Aging Society, 2003). Older adults who are obese are more likely to suffer from persistent and chronic symptoms of illness, and to report symptoms of depression. In addition to having difficulty with activities of daily living, older obese adults are more likely to not be able to walk very far, go shopping, or participate in other activities that enrich our lives (Center on an Aging Society).

EPILOGUE

Does our culture truly appreciate and admire those who have all that comes with living a long full life? Who cares? You may read dozens of magazine articles celebrating the vitality of the aged, but you won't see one ad like this in any of those publications: *"Lacking Experience and Wisdom? Want to Look Older so People Will Respect You? Try Our New Aging Cream for Instant Wrinkles and Gray Hair."*

I'm not worried about my future. If I get to the point that nobody wants to hire me, marry me, love me, if it takes me even longer to remember your name, if all my hair turns white, and if I have no idea what young people are thinking about, I'll still have one option open to me: I can always write another book... and I'll STILL be looking fine and feeling good while I'm doing it. AMEN!

References

Arteburn, D., Craine, P., & Sullivan, S. (2004). The coming epidemic of obesity in elderly Americans. Journal of the American Geriatric Society, 52, 1907-1912.

Baranoski, S. (2001). Skin tears. Nurse Manager, 32, 25-31.

Bouchard, C., (1989). Genetic factors in obesity. Medical Clinics of North America, 73(1), 67-81.

Brockman, G., Tsaih, S., Neuschi. C., Churchill, G., & Li, R. (November 4, 2008). Genetic factors contributing to obesity and body weight can act through mechanisms affecting muscle weight, fat weight or both. Physiological Genomics, 10, 1152.

Brown, J., Wimpenny, P., & Maughan, H. (2004). Skin problems in people with obesity. Nursing Standard, 18, 38-42.

Center on an Aging Society (2003). Obesity among older Americans. Retrieved July 23, 2013, from http://ihcrp.georgetown.edu/agingsociety/pdfs/obesity2.pdf

Corpas, E., Harman, S., & Blackman, M., (1993). Human growth hormone and human aging. Endocrinology Review, 14, 20-39

Daniels, J. (2006). Obesity: America's epidemic. American Journal of Nursing, 106, 40-9.

Department of Health and Human Services (2000). Healthy people 2010: Understanding and improving health. (2nd ed.). Washington, DC: U.S. Government Printing Office.

Dick, J.J. (2004). Weight loss interventions for adult obesity: Evidence for practice Worldviews On Evidence-Based Nursing / Sigma Theta Tau International, Honor Society of Nursing, 1(4), 209-214.

Donini, L., Chumlea, W., Vellas, B., del Balzo, V., & Cannalla, C. (2006). Aging Health. 2, 47-51. Retrieved August 2, 2013, from www.futuremedicine.com.doi/abs/

Federal Interagency Forum on Aging (2006). Older Americans update 2006: Key indicators of well-being. Retrieved July 28, 2013, from www.aginastats.gov/agingstats.net/

Flood, M., & Newman, A. (2007). Obesity in older adults: Synthesis of findings and recommendations for clinical practice. Journal of Gerontological Nursing, 33, 19-35.

Gary, P., Hunt, W., Koehler, K., & VanderJagt, B. (1992). Longitudinal study of dietary intakes and plasma lipids in healthy elderly men and women. American Journal of Clinic Nutrition, 55,682-688.

Glass, T., Rasmussen, M., & Schwartz, B. (2006). Neighborhoods and obesity in older adults: The Baltimore memory study. American Journal of Preventive Medicine, 31(6), 455-463. Retrieved August 1, 2013 from: www.pubmedcentral.nih.gov/articlerender.

Grundy, S. (2004). Obesity, metabolic syndrome, cardiovascular disease. The Journal of Clinical Endocrinology & Metabolism. 89, 2595-2600.

Hanna, I. & Wenger, N. (2005). Secondary prevention of coronary heart disease in elderly patients. American Family Physician, 7, 2209-2296. Retrieved August 1, 2013, from www.aafp.org/afp/2005615/2289.html

Hu, F., Li, T., Colditz, G., Willett, W., & Manson, J. (2003). Television watching and other Sedentary behaviors, in relation to risk of obesity and type 2 diabetes mellitus in women. JAMA, 289, 1785-1791.

Karlson, E., Mandl, L., Aweh, G., Sangha, O., Liang, M., & Grodstein, F. (2003). Total hip replacement due to osteoarthritis: The importance of age, obesity, and other modifiable risk factors. American Journal of Medicine,114, 93-98.

Leveille, S., Wee, C., & Iezzoni, L. (2005). Trends in obesity and arthritis among baby boomers and their predecessors 1971-2002. American Journal of Public Health, 95(9), 1607-1613.

Lorig, K., & Fries, J. (2006). The arthritis helpbook, 6th ed. Reading, MA: Perseus.

Lorig, K., , H., Sobel, D., Laurent, D., Gonzalez, V., & Minor, M. (2006). Living a healthy life with chronic conditions 3rd ed. Boulder, CO: Bull.
Move Forward
http://www.moveforwardpt.com/Resources/Detail.aspx?cid=c44b7f87-e37c-4274-9cd8-5f2a79c9129e

National blueprint: Increasing physical activity among adults aged 50 and older. (n.d.). Retrieved July 26, 2013from www.agingblueprint.org/

National Digestive Diseases Information Clearinghouse (2004). Gallstones. Retrieved August 15, 2008, from http://digestive.nidd.nih.gov/ddiseases/pubs/gallstones/index.htm#causes

Newman, A. (2002). Patient teaching tools and self-help techniques: Focus on cultural diversity. In Luggen, A. & Meiner, S (Eds.)., Care of Arthritis in the Older Adult. NY: Springer.

NIH Publication No. 01-3680 (2006). Understanding adult obesity. Retrieved July 28, 2013 from, http://win.niddk.gov/publications/understanding.htm
Obesity among older Americans
http://www.aging.senate.gov/crs/aging3.pdf

Patterson, R., Frank, L., Kristal, A., & White, E. (2004). A comprehensive examination of health conditions associated with obesity in older adults. American Journal of Preventive Medicine, 27, 385-390.

Resnick, B. (2001). Managing arthritis with exercise. Geriatric Nursing, 22(3), 143-150.

Sweeney, C., Blair, C., Anderson, K., Lazovich, D. & Folsom, A. (2004). Risk factors for breast cancer in elderly women. American Journal of Epidemiology, 160, 868-875.

Tabloski, P. (2006). The respiratory system. Gerontological Nursing. (pp. 460-516. Upper Saddle River, NJ: Pearson Prentice Hall.

Tucker, S. (2006). Nutrition and aging. In PA Tabloski (Ed.) Gerontological Nursing. (pp. 110-154). Upper Saddle River, NJ: Pearson Prentice Hall.

U.S. Department of Health and Human Services. (n.d.). Healthy people 2010. Retrieved January 26, 2009 from: www.healthypeople.gov/

Vainio, H., & Bianchini, F (Eds.).(2002). IARC handbooks of cancer prevention Vol. 6: Weight control and physical activity. Lyon, France: IARC Press.

Villareal, D., Apovian, C., Kushner, R., & Klein, S. (2005). Obesity in older adults: technical Review and position statement of the American Society for Nutrition and NAASO, The Obesity Society. American Journal of Clinical Nutrition,82(5), 923-934. Retrieved July 29, 2013,from www.ajcn.org/cgi/content/full/82/5/923 .

Wallace, J., Schulte, W., Nakeeb, A., & Andris, D. (2003). Health problems related to severe obesity. Retrieved July 24, 2013, from http://healthlink.mcw.edu/article/984434798.html

Wilson, P., & Kannel (2007). Obesity, diabetes, and risk of cardiovascular disease in the elderly. The American Journal of Geriatric Cardiology, 11, 119-124.

World Health Organization (2005). Global strategy on diet, physical activity, and health. Retrieved July 29, 2013, from www.who.int/dietphysicalactivity/publications/facts/obesity/en/

Yan, L.L, Daviglus, M.L., Liu, K., Pirzada, A., Garside, D.B., Schiffer, L., et al. (2004). Body mass index and health-related quality of life in adults 65 years and older. Obesity Research, 12, 69-76.

Zerah, F., Harf, A., Perlemuter, L., Lorino, H., Lorino, A., & Atlan, G. (1993). Effects of obesity on respiratory resistance. Chest, 103, 1470-1476.